# UP THE DOWNHILL SLIDE

JOAN RHINER VON LEHE

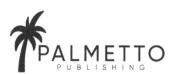

PALMETTO
PUBLISHING

Charleston, SC
www.PalmettoPublishing.com

Up the Downhill Slide

ISBN: 978-1-64990-406-5

# DEDICATION

To the grandest of grands — Norah, Drew, James, and Reed.  You are my inspiration for finding pleasure in growing old.  My heart overflows.

# CONTENTS

# ACKNOWLEDGEMENTS

Although rewarding, writing a book is certainly no piece of cake. It is a world brimming with details, overthinking, and countless frustrations . . . yet I regard it as a luring challenge with intense gratification.

I simply could not have completed this project without the help of my loving daughters, Rebecca and Laura. Their willingness to read, and reread . . . so many times, means the world. I am delighted that they remembered what they learned in English class, unlike their mother. Their input on phrasing and grammar pretty much saved me. And typos? Let's just say that proofreading my own manuscript did not work. Most importantly, I thank them from the bottom of my heart for their patience, support, and encouragement. To show my appreciation, I promised that I would make my "downhill slide" a great source of entertainment while living out our real-time drama, "As the Tables Turn." I can only hope they remember that I took great pride in caring for them . . . and that love and laughter go hand in hand.

After sending my girls a few too many emails with false promises of a "final" manuscript, I assured them that I would have another pair of eyes critique my "actual" final manuscript. My dear friend, Melissa Ellenburg, graciously agreed to proofread for me. I am more than grateful for her willingness to assist . . . and for her feeling "honored" to do so.

# INTRODUCTION

Life has taught me many lessons through the years. The older I get, the more I learn — the hard way, of course. I think I have finally realized that facts are facts, and some things you just can't change no matter how hard you try. That has not stopped me from fighting a good fight and trying my best to defy the odds. It is just my rebellious nature. I do not like to brag, but it only took me two months to tackle the issues that the aging process has so graciously introduced me to recently — and I use the word "tackle" loosely.

In case you haven't noticed, aging is inevitable; therefore, it is with great pleasure that I offer this short, daily journal to make jumping through the hoops and over the hurdles of senior citizenship a bit more tolerable. It's all about attitude. I plan to enjoy the gift of old age the best way I know how. It is a privilege that has been denied to many. A little mildly insane behavior can go a long way toward making the most of growing old and enjoying the ride. The way I see it, old age is a great excuse to act crazy . . . well, craziER. I feel as though I have gained "permission" to become a not-so-run-of-the-mill geriatric inhabitant. My time has arrived.

No doubt, there will be many new challenges coming our way as we "ripen" with age. This enlightening journal is packed full of priceless information, ideas, solutions, and such . . . sort of. Proceed with caution. You will read of a few truths, some half-truths, but mostly a lot of overactive thought processes in my personal attempt to prepare myself for life's inescapable decline. I'm glad to share. Happy aging!

# FIFTY SHADES OF GRAY

This morning, I looked in the mirror. I can't believe it didn't crack. Once upon a time, I was decent-looking, but my good features have drifted far away into never-never land and left the not-so-good ones to stand out like a neon sign in the black of night. I'm in dire need of improvement to my looks. I realize that my options are limited since there is not much to work with. My hair I can help . . . the rest, not so much. Well, that's not altogether a true statement. This "image in the mirror" can't really help her hair at all. She's doing well to brush it. She must leave the rest to a professional. A few weeks ago, she left the salon with enough confidence to enter as a contestant in the upcoming, local Ms. Senior Pageant at the civic center. She was stunning . . . well, at least from the neck up. But as soon as she slept on her hair, it looked like she stuck her finger in a light socket. So, she wet it down and tamed it with gel. Then she looked like she had been slimed. So much for the beauty pageant. And now that a few weeks have passed, every strand of hair on her head seems to be turning a different color — mostly shades of gray. What is her natural color anyway? She has no idea! Unfortunately, her drastic, two-toned part has earned her the nickname, "Skunk!" And a point to ponder: is this "pitiful reflection" the only one that worries about dying at the right time? Croaking that is. She really hopes it happens right after she gets her hair done. She's not so sure that she would trust a corpse cosmetologist to make her look good for her entrance into the pearly gates.

Note to self: Call Jennifer to make a hair appointment — pronto!

# THE MASK

Today is World Sleep Day. That's a new one on me. I do believe that there is a day to celebrate anything and everything, and some are just ridiculous — like National Crayon Day or World Naked Gardening Day. But World Sleep Day is beyond a great idea. I'd like to personally commend whoever thought up this one. I wonder if my boss would mind if I stayed in bed and did not go to work today? I just don't have the energy I used to have when I was young. It's a downright effort to go to work these days. Maybe I could at least show up late and say that I had just been diagnosed with narcolepsy. That way, if I happened to nod off with my head resting on the keyboard, he would not ask me about the little, square imprints on my face. That reminds me . . . I have quite a variety of eye masks to share with anyone else who would like to celebrate this day of sleep that commemorates one-third of our lives. I believe I'll pack them up and offer them to my co-workers who may be interested in participating in this awesome "holiday." Not only do the masks block out the light, but they are also cute. My favorite one says, "Leave me alone." It is very effective, for more than one reason. Not only does it keep out the light, but it serves as a silent and emphatic version of "I have a headache," which is very important these days.

Note to self: Update resume, and pray I do not need a divorce attorney.

# CELEBRATE GREEN

Happy St. Patty's Day! I may be old, but I still love to celebrate holidays. I am wearing my green today so that I will not get pinched . . . and hopefully, I will not pinch myself when I am putting on my green spandex. I love all shades of green, so I love that there is a day to celebrate it. My mother-in-law had Irish in her blood, so I always think of her fondly on this day. Because of her, I always made sure my kids wore something to show off their "Quinlan" Irish heritage. We had a little, felt leprechaun that I proudly pinned on my older daughter each year on this day, which was a gift from her Grammy for her very first St. Patrick's Day. A few years later, we acquired a plastic, green heart with gold letters that said, "I'm Irish." My younger daughter wore it each March 17th. I am not into fashion, so I just drank green beer. I don't remember that it ever brought me good luck, but that didn't keep me from trying. Shamrocks and rainbows didn't bring me much luck either, for that matter. But all of that could change today. It is five o'clock somewhere, and I am way past due for some good luck. Here's to celebrating Irish culture and pursuing my search for a pot of gold. May I never be too old to celebrate. Cheers!

Note to self: Buy beer, green food coloring, and a lottery ticket.

# MY "AHA!" MOMENT

I helped throw a bridal shower today at church for a close family friend. I served the punch. Everyone has learned that it is best not to put me on the decorating or food committee. Serving punch is relatively risk free. I always volunteer for clean-up duty as well. That is usually safe. It was a good day. The only thing I managed to break was a plastic ladle. As I took a gander at the lovely gifts that were displayed, it occurred to me that those of us who have been married "forever" should deservingly be eligible for an "anniversary shower." We have been using the same CorningWare for decades, and it just gets old looking at the outdated Cornflower Blue and Spice of Life patterns. Appliances and such have also greatly improved on looks and quality through the years, not to mention the fact that my dishes look like they have been used for plate-spinning practice. The chips and cracks are massive. Yes, I would love to donate all my old stuff and start over. I think we deserve a reward for growing old with someone and staying married all these years. A lightbulb just went off in my head. I believe that maybe I will start a new trend with the anniversary shower idea. Well, there is no "maybe" to it. I'm going for it.

Note to self: Buy invitations, and make anniversary shower guest list.

# MARCH 19

# QUACK, QUACK

I attended a seminar on workplace violence today. We had a three-hour class conducted by a police officer telling us how to protect ourselves in case of an emergency or threatening situation. We were encouraged to have a plan in case an employee went "postal." Really? Whatever happened to having a good ole temper tantrum? The theme and motto of the seminar was, "Run, Hide, Fight!" Well, number one, I can't run because I have bad knees. Number two, I was never good at hide-and-seek, so hopefully, squatting beneath my desk would be a clever enough barricade. At least I'm smart enough not to stand in front of a window. And fight? I have no problem with taking off my shoe and bopping someone over the head. There was one semi-helpful suggestion though. We were reminded that we should turn off our cell phones in order to avoid giving away our location in case it went off. I expounded upon that idea and proposed a scheme to change the ringtone to a quacking duck, toss the phone into the hall, then borrow someone's phone to call it so that the shooter would turn his attention to the noisy, feathery fowl. I suggested that a better plan would be called, "Walk, Squat, Distract!" Being the oldest one in the class, my "older and wiser" bits of wisdom were confidently verbalized. I don't think the instructor was too impressed with my input. Bottom line, my suggestion went over like a lead balloon.

Note to self: Get someone to help me move my desk into the vault.

MARCH 20

# THE I-DON'T-CARE-ABOUT-MEDICARE SYNDROME

Medicare is just around the corner. Yippee!! I have less than six months until I reach this glorious milestone, and I am already being flooded with phone calls, mail, and emails . . . and not just about Medicare. I am drowning in information on funeral insurance, walk-in tubs, oxygen tanks, memory repair, blood pressure meds, reverse mortgage, senior dating websites, aging skin, Alzheimer's prevention — you name it. Like I really need a reminder that I will be six feet under sooner than later. I also find it amusing that the very next email is one that offers information about pain management, alcohol rehab, or something along those lines. Go figure! And if I hear about one more webinar on senior benefits assistance programs, I think I will scream. Coverage gaps, part A, part B, part C, part D, advantage plans, supplements, etc. Grrr! Last, but not least, I have absolutely NO desire to attend a seminar to learn about donut holes. I love the ones at the bakery, and that's all that matters.

Note to self: Call about renewing pain meds. Go to the bakery for donuts.

# THE COVER-UP

What is it with aging and lack of sleep? I woke up at least three times last night, and each time it took longer to go back to sleep. The first time was because my indigestion was so bad that I could not figure out whether or not I was having a heart attack. After knocking the jar of Tums off the nightstand, I finally found them by feeling around on the floor. Naturally, the lid was not on tight, so they went everywhere. I managed to find two, blew the dust bunnies off, chewed them, and was able to ease on back to sleep. Then, of course, an hour later I had to get up to pee. I nearly knocked my shoulder off as I ran into the door frame because it was pitch black in my room. Evidently, the night light found its way out of the plug and onto the counter, again. Then I fell into the toilet because someone left the seat up, again. After drying off my bottom, I crawled back into the bed, but by the time I untwisted all the covers, I was wide awake from practically having to remake the bed. When I finally dozed off again, the garbage truck decided to come at 4 a.m., and the noise was ... well, noisy. It doesn't appear that sleeping soundly will ever be an option again. I'm just plain tired, and I don't see it improving with age. The bags under my eyes are a dead giveaway. As much makeup as I use to try to hide them, I am investigating buying stock in Cover Girl.

Note to self: Order a case of concealer.

# FITNESS OR FATNESS?

I'm looking over today's mail, and I keep getting these flyers about the new fitness center in town. I feel honored that they want me as a member. I am really thinking about joining and gracing them with my presence, but the idea of me showing up in exercise pants and a tank top has me backing off the idea a little … well, a lot. They would likely have to give out nausea pills to their members as soon as I walked in the door since my rolls of flab pretty much confirm that I am related to the Michelin Tire man. Plus, the bat wings on my upper arms would likely send me flying across the gym if I moved them up and down too fast while doing my jumping jacks. I suppose I should not be concerned about all that. I should just be concerned about my physical well-being. I could stand to drop a few pounds, and cardio health is without a doubt on the forefront of my brain at this stage of the game. However, it would be cheaper just to hop on the treadmill that serves as a clothes rack in my basement. I'll need to consider this a wee bit longer. It will just take some more thought.

Note to self: Lie on couch, eat bonbons, and wait for the next fitness flyer to come in the mail.

# SAY "SQUEEZE"

Today was my lucky day.  It was time, once again, for my yearly mammogram.  Whoopee!!  Somewhere along the line, I got the idea that when I got older, I would not have to get squashed and photographed every year.  I guess wishful thinking does not always work.  It just never gets any easier to go through this "drama-trauma" experience.  To start off, I forgot that you are not supposed to have on deodorant when you are having your boob picture made, so after nearly wiping myself raw with a washcloth, I slipped on the little robe.  Of course, as soon as I figured out how to put it on, the tech pulled it off on one side and proceeded to lift and flop my boob up on the cold, metal platform.  Once I caught my breath, I got to watch the humongous machine lower on me like a boulder falling off a mountain.  Then I was instructed to hold my breath and not to move ... like I could really go anywhere.  Oh, the joys of woman-hood never seem to end.  You would think at my age the doctors would give me a break from such torture.  But no.  On the way out, I was handed an appointment card for next year.

Note to self:  Buy Advil, and cancel next year's appointment.

# IT'S ALL ABOUT IMAGE

What's all the hype about crocheting these days?  It seems to be making a comeback in a big way.  All my friends are grooving on their multi-colored yarn and crochet hooks.  Boring!  I think it would make me crazier than a bedbug, even more nuts than I already am.  And I can't afford to pull out my hair.  It's thinning enough on its own as it is.  The little baby blankets are adorable, but that's why we have stores.  I couldn't even sit still long enough to finish a row.  And to me, to watch someone sitting there crocheting epitomizes the portrayal of an old lady.  I'm trying very hard to stay away from that.  My image needs to be one of youth.  Let's see.  Just picture me in a flight suit standing in front of a plane.  Oh wait, I'm afraid of flying.  Hmm, maybe a better image would be to stand on a tennis court with a racquet in my hand.  Maybe not.  Stiff muscles and arthritis make it difficult to return a ball.  How about standing on a beach with a surfboard?  Now there is an image that would suit me.  I love the beach.  Speaking of suit . . . I wonder if wet suits come in 3XL?

Note to self:  Order book:  *Crocheting for Dummies.*

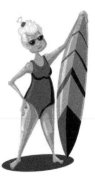

# BEHIND THE 8 BALL

The topic at my house over the weekend was downsizing. I've been batting this idea back and forth for a while now. Having mixed emotions about this subject is quite the under-statement. Where would I start? It would take me decades to go through all my junk and decide what I needed to keep and what I could do without. I am not a materialistic person, but I am emotionally attached to my belongings. Sentimental is good, right? There are many things that I do not use often, but when I need them, I need them. Practical is good, right? I have way too much to clean, and I just don't have the energy anymore. I can't see well anyway, so what will an inch or two of dust hurt, right? Things that have been in my family forever will likely be sold or tossed out when I am gone, and I just can't bear that thought. So, I need to keep an eye on them for as long as I can, right? When I can't use the stairs any longer, I will just buy one of those chairs that ride up and down the bannister. That sounds kind of fun, right? And I like fun. Okay, I need to be practical . . . yet I need to follow my heart. What to do, what to do?

Note to self: Go to Walmart, buy Magic 8 Ball, and pray it does not land on "REPLY HAZY."

# READ THE DOTS

I just hate not being able to see. Why does eyesight have to be on the list of deteriorating abilities when you surpass your middle-aged years? It's the most important of our senses by far. And I do know for a fact that it only gets worse with age. Otherwise, why would my mother call the bank and ask for her bank statements to come in braille? Speaking of braille, at least all the nameplates outside our offices at work have the person's name and department written in braille underneath the printing. I just hope nobody sees me trying to rub my fingertips raw. And ask me how thrilled I am that my eye doctor recently told me I have the beginning of cataracts. The eyedrop regimen alone would be too much of a challenge for me. And chalk another one up to genetics — macular degeneration runs in my family. Just imagine having a big, cloudy blob right in the middle of what you are looking at. I guess that it could be an advantage if my husband were to get a case of deteriorating looks before I do. I am learning that I can usually find a bright side to everything.

Note to self: Buy salve for fingertips, and learn braille.

# A NEW KIND OF RV

I've always dreamed of living in one of those swanky retirement villages. A swimming pool year-round, golf courses at my disposal, and entertainment on the square every night. I could join yoga classes, arts and crafts classes, and bridge clubs. I think that it would just suit me to a "T." I wouldn't even have to cook or clean if I didn't want to. That would be the cherry on top. Well, now that I am technically eligible to be a resident, I am having second thoughts. Suddenly, I am visualizing myself cruising around in a golf cart trying to make my way to the med clinic without getting run over by another golf cart with a less-than-qualified driver. And I am quite sure there would be dirty old men trying to flirt with me at the ice cream shop. Eww! I would also be willing to bet that the local beauty salon would attempt to experiment with their craft by turning us old ladies' different shades of purplish-blue on a weekly basis. Lastly, going to the "in-activity" center is not exactly my idea of a senile haven. Playing card games and checkers would bore me to tears. Why is dreaming about something always better than really having it happen? I have a feeling that life will not be as exciting at the retirement village as I had envisioned.

Note to self: Brush up on Old Maid card game and checkers.

# PLUMBING LEAKS

Today, I saw an ad on TV for a new-and-improved brand of incontinence pads. I am not quite there yet, but then again, I know that the everything-is-in-working-order days are on the decline. Occasionally, a simple sneeze or a belly laugh will be an indicator of that sad and upcoming fact of life. I'm sure it will cut down on more activities than I ever imagined. For instance, sitting through long movies at the theatre will likely become an issue. It's not like I can put the movie on pause while I go pee. And what if I get stuck in traffic? I can't carry around a coffee can just in case I get struck with an uncontrollable urge to relieve myself. But what would I do? And what if I go square dancing and hop a little too hard on the landing? Am I just supposed to promenade around the puddle on the floor? And what about horse-back riding? Forget it! These scenarios swimming around in my head prompted me to pay attention to the ad. TENA pads will be my new best friend. I vow to remain active in my old age, so bring on the music and let the "TENA Twist" begin.

Note to self: Clean out closet to make room for bulk shipment of TENA pads.

MARCH 29

# OFF TO THE RACES

I went to the local medical equipment store today just to browse. Getting old certainly is more appealing than it used to be, if I had to guess. There were all kinds of new-fangled, assist-me-with-whatever aids. I mainly looked at walking aids because my knees were practically screaming aloud for help. I was amazed at the variety of items available. Wooden canes and stripped-down walker models are a thing of the past. Now there are canes in all shapes, sizes, and colors. One prong, two prongs, three prongs, four prongs, canes with shock absorbers, and canes that fold up. I was like a kid in a toy store. I want the designer cane with pink flowers that I spotted. I'll add it to my birthday list. The walkers came with wheels, without wheels, with baskets, without baskets, with seats, without seats. The options were limitless. One can even buy accessories for them, such as caddies, trays, and cup holders. Personally, I'm holding out for a motorized cart. Much more fun. Not sure what color I want, though. I will need a cup holder for sure . . . you know, for happy hour. I wonder if they have walker and cart races at the retirement village? I'll order padded hand grips with streamers just in case.

Note to self: Put walker/cart race idea in suggestion box. Buy helmet.

# MENTALLY FIT

I have always read and heard that doing crossword puzzles and playing word games will help deter cognitive decline in elderly folks. I certainly hope it's true because I have been playing word games all my life. I don't do number games though. Sudoku is nothing short of maddening because I don't like numbers. I am envisioning a fit of rage just thinking about it. Supposedly, there has not actually been enough evidence that either have helped to slow the chances of developing dementia. I figured it cannot hurt, so I ordered a case of easy, large-print word puzzle books. I just hope they have the answers in the back. I read this morning that high intelligence in childhood is a strong shield against cognitive decline. Well, you can't believe everything you read. I plan to stay mentally active until the end of my days. I know eventually that Bingo will be my main avenue for staying mentally active. I just hope they use picture Bingo cards at the retirement village. No numbers for me. Hmm, another idea to drop in the suggestion box. The social director may be sorry she ever met me.

Note to self: Find out childhood IQ.

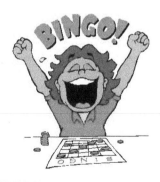

MARCH 31

# TRASH AND TREASURES

Today, I started cleaning out closets to make room for my bulk shipment of TENA pads. I made three piles. One was "stuff to keep", one was "stuff to throw away", and one was "stuff to donate." The "stuff to keep" pile was sizably larger than the other two piles. I just have trouble getting rid of things. I finally talked myself into adding a few more items to the "stuff to donate" pile. I quickly put them in the car before I had time to change my mind, and off I went to the thrift store. I took them to the counter to get a receipt for the items I reluctantly donated. A few things caught my eye while waiting, so I decided just to browse around the store for a bit. The old saying, "One man's trash is another man's treasure," is so true. I found some fantastic bargains. I made my purchases rather quickly so that I could get the car unloaded before dark.

Note to self: Cancel bulk shipment of TENA pads.

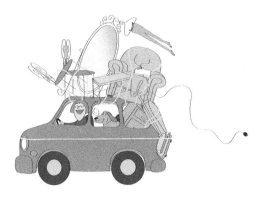

# LOSING FRIENDS

April Fools' Day is here at last. I love to pull pranks, so today was especially fun. It's important to laugh. Socializing and having fun with friends will keep me young. Well, if not, I will die trying. I spent the morning conjuring up some practical jokes to play on my friends. I was at my neighbor's house just before lunch, and while she was outside watering her plants, I decided to "short-sheet" her bed. Nothing like crawling into bed exhausted and not being able to stretch your legs out. Wish I could be a fly on the wall. This afternoon when our CLP (Cognitive Loss Prevention) group met, we were playing Tiddlywinks, and I decided to swap out Ethel's white wine for lemon juice when she got up to pee. It was quite a rude awakening and well worth the laugh, even though she spewed it all over Ruby when she spit it out. Irene was nothing short of perturbed when she could not find her plate of food that she set down. I moved it to another room. Hide and seek is so fun, at least when I am the one doing the hiding. When we sat back down to play a game of Go Fish, the look on Beulah's face was hilarious as she sat on the whoopee cushion. I made sure the fun would continue into the night. I wonder how long it took Vera to find the pictures I rearranged on her walls. Last, but not least, I hope Matilda does not toss her cookies when she sees the fake vomit I left on her front porch.

Note to self: Remind my ex-friends that laughter is good medicine.

# SAY WHAT?

Today was downright depressing after having so much fun yesterday. I wonder if mood swings count as exercise. I'll check into it. Depression runs in my family, so I need to try my best to beat it . . . especially since I am aging, which is depressing in and of itself. I have read that taking a class or volunteering helps to ward off depression. Volunteering sounds a little too much like work, so I called the local junior college today to see what classes were available for senior citizens. A dance class and a computer class were both being offered the next semester. The only way I would take the computer class is if they furnished jumbo keyboards, so that was not an option. That left dance class. Learning new moves could be fun. Fun is always at the top of my list. When I showed up for class, I was very surprised . . . and disappointed. It was a ballroom dance class. I thought the lady said, "barroom dance." Fortunately, it did not cost me a penny to drop the class.

Note to self: Inquire about Miracle Ear.

# APRIL 3

# PASTIMES

Since the dance class did not work out, I needed to find another constructive way to pass the time. I was in search of a new hobby. My life coach suggested that I learn a new skill. This would be tough. I already know how to do so many things. I googled learning new skills online. I did not want any more surprises like the dance class debacle. There were all sorts of crazy ideas. Culinary arts — you couldn't pay me. Pet care — I already know how to walk the dog and feed the cat. Speaking and translating other languages — I took two years of Spanish in high school…dos años. Public speaking — I doubt they offer babbling skills, which will soon be my language of choice. Knitting — knitting needles are a dangerous weapon, and I don't trust myself. Bartending — again, I don't trust myself. Bodybuilding — that will be impossible to do from my lift chair. Yada-yada-yada.

Note to self:  Find new life coach.

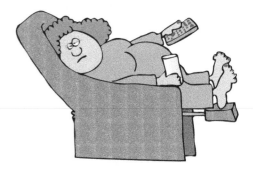

APRIL 4

# FUN IN THE SUN

I can't quit yawning. I am nearly suffering from exhaustion because of all the reading and studying I'm having to do regarding old people dilemmas. It's practically a full-time job. Vitamin D deficiency is just one of about 500 issues that will more than likely intrude on my well-being as a senior citizen. Being elderly is the first risk factor listed for this condition. Well, that's great to know. There's not a lot I can do about that. How encouraging. Moving on to the symptoms. Fatigue and tiredness are listed first. Really? That could be attributed to a gazillion other things as well, so it's all just a guess as far as I'm concerned. The article also said that exposing your skin to sunlight and eating fish may reduce the risk of vitamin D deficiency. So, since I do not eat fish, I will at least make a bold effort to get more sun.

Note to self: Buy skimpy swimsuit for added sun exposure. Patch holes in privacy fence.

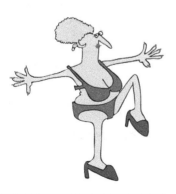

# MOUTH GONE SOUTH

My morning started off with my annual trip to the dentist . . . or at least I think I went last year. I was escorted to the chair, and the assistant pinned the little bib on me. The thought crossed my mind that the bib-on-a-chain would be nice to have when I get to the nursing home. Drool can surely make a mess. I was nearly dozing off when the hygienist pointed that annoying, overhead lamp in my face. Then the scraping began. It felt and sounded like she was scraping cement. I knew that plaque build-up gets worse with age, but I thought that was just in your arteries. I've never had teeth issues until recently. As soon as I entered my sixth decade, I had to have all my fillings replaced because they were old and worn out. A few months later, I had two molars crack, resulting in a new set of crowns. Not the kind of crowns I had always dreamed of. Then I had the beginning of gum disease, so I had to have my gums deep cleaned. Ouch! Not recommended. Today, when the cleaning was done, the dentist checked my mouth and explained that as I age, my teeth will shift, become more discolored, become sensitive due to receding gums, and will undergo worn-down enamel. I don't think they will be asking me to model for their "Signature Smile" brochure as I had hoped. Time is running out for my claim to fame.

Note to self: Start saving money for dentures. Contact denture company about modeling for their brochure cover.

# PILL THRILL

I went to the pharmacy today and purchased a gigantic weekly pill container. My meds are becoming too numerous to count. I take a blue pill to alleviate symptoms brought on by the white one. Then one of those will cause another issue, so I take a yellow one to fix it. Then if I develop a new symptom, I take a different white one. I have several doctors, and each one has prescribed several medicines. I don't know what kind of pill I'm taking for what ailment. It gets confusing. Now, I can just read the labels that tell me how many to take a day and drop them in my cute, new flip-top pill holder. If I know what day of the week it is, I will take the correct pills. I keep a calendar in the kitchen and mark the day with an "X" if it has come and gone. Most of the time, I remember to mark it. And if I forget to take my pills the day before, I can just take both days at once to make up for it. My new pill container will help me keep it all straight.

Note to self: Put 911 on speed dial.

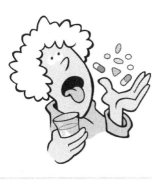

# FLOWER POWER

It is just now beginning to feel like spring, and I am past ready. The winter was cold. Ask my bones. I just function better when it's warm — mentally and physically. Today, I piddled in the garden trying to get my flower beds ready for spring flowers. I just love flowers. They can brighten my mood, even on a bad day. I select most of them for their names. Nothing like marigolds to make me feel merry, dandelions to make me feel dandy, and gladiolus to make me glad. I will not be buying any bleeding hearts or spider mums. I spent the afternoon picking weeds and cleaning the leaves, sticks, and debris from the beds. I know not to plant bulbs again. Mine did not come up last year, and I can't dig them up because I don't remember where I put them. The sunshine felt so good beating down on me, but when my scalp felt like it was on fire, I had to go in. The top of my head was fried, and I was covered in dirt . . . but it will all be worth it in the end. The neighbors will be so impressed and green with envy when they see the "Yard of the Month" sign in my yard.

Note to self: Make "Yard of the Month" sign. Buy aloe, sun hat, and Rogaine for Women.

APRIL 8

# AFTERNOON DELIGHT

All my doctors seem to agree that fiber is very important, especially as we age. So, I decided to shop for fiber supplements. I went to the pharmacy and read labels so that I could make the best decision about what to buy. I barely got out of the store before closing time, and I got there at noon. There was a whole aisle full of options. Metamucil, Benefiber, Fiber Cleanse, Citrucel, Fiber Choice, Psyllium Husk, Fitness Fiber, UniFiber, Triple Fiber, Fiber Smart, Fiber Advance, Bio-Fiber — and that's not all of them. My favorite name was Fiber Delight. Really? Dairy Delight I can understand. Ice cream is to die for — but fiber? And in my opinion, it should be against the law to make so many kinds. There were powders, granules, pills, capsules, chewable tablets, and gummies — in every flavor under the sun. Green apple, wild berry, orange, lemon, grape, cherry. I felt like I was on the Kool-Aid aisle. I had to remind myself that I was shopping for "eat and go" products. I can't wait to try all the flavors. By midday every day, I'll be feeling like a champ. Afternoon delight will now have a whole new meaning.

Note to self: Take Fiber every evening. Don't schedule any morning appointments.

# TRIAL AND ERROR

Since purchasing my new Fiber Delight gummies, I have had to consider purchasing adult protective underwear. Off to the pharmacy one more time. They will know me on a first name basis by the end of the week. Once again, too many choices. Medtronics, Fit Right, Wellness Briefs, Abena, Pro Care, Tranquility, North Shore, Attends, Prevail, Reassure, and of course, Depends. I think my favorite was Crinklz Briefs adult printed diapers. Yes, they crinkle when you walk . . . I guess so you cannot sneak off while trying to escape the premises? Another favorite was the Safari prints by Rearz. Like I'm going to be sashaying around in one trying to look cute. I do think they should at least win the clever name prize. Then I had to pick a style: pull-on or tabs. And there were several absorbency choices as well. Well, I do believe I am smart enough not to choose "light" and take a chance. No thanks! I don't really want to hear them announce, "Cleanup on aisle four."

Note to self: Buy sample packs to test. Stay home for two weeks.

# APRIL 10

# BROKEN THERMOSTAT

I truly thought that I had surpassed the age for hot flashes. It appears that they will be never-ending. Out of nowhere, here one came. Last night, I had to get up, take off my PJ bottoms, take off my long-sleeve shirt, and change into a thin, short-sleeve T-shirt. By this time, I was wide awake. Click! Click! I turned the ceiling fan from low to high, and it sounded like a helicopter was preparing for flight. I stood directly beneath it for several minutes trying to cool off. As my body thermostat attempted to adjust, I slowly began to feel a little more comfortable as I prayed the fan blades would not come flying off the thirty-year-old, wobbly contraption overhead. As my body temperature went down, I finally dozed off to sleep, only to wake up freezing as the fan blew across the sweat beads all over my body. Then I had to get up, turn the fan back down to low, and put the covers back on. Repeat. Repeat. Repeat.

Note to self: Buy new ceiling fan with remote control. Purchase Estroven caplets.

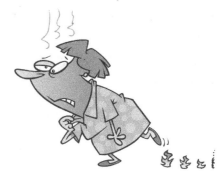

# DISCOUNT DILEMMAS

I have always heard that one advantage of getting old is that you can get senior discounts. Well, I'm all about saving a dime. So, I went online and printed off a list of where I could take advantage of the senior discounts. All kinds of restaurants, grocery stores, motels, department stores, movie theaters, and fast food joints were listed. Some give a 10% discount, some give a free drink, some give smaller sizes for less money, etc. The problem is, not all locations "participate." Well, that's a bunch of garbage. It's much easier for the employees just to say that. I guess they figure seniors will take them at their word. Not this senior! Their managers may just get an earful if I don't get the discount I have rightfully earned. They also have made it complicated because they all have different rules. I will have to write out an itinerary for the week because some places only offer discounts on certain days. On top of that, some establishments consider seniors to be 55 and older, some 60 and older, some 62 and older, and some 65 and older. How about a little consistency here folks! Just because we get confused easily doesn't mean they should take advantage of the fact.

Note to self: Write to AARP about senior discount confusion. Buy giant calculator to add up savings.

# SLEEP-DEPRIVED

I am really dragging today. I did not sleep well at all last night, again. It took me forever to go to sleep because I was mentally mapping out my trek all over town to check out the senior discounts that I was due. When I finally got to sleep, I suddenly woke up at 1:23 a.m. with big, red numbers staring at me. When I saw 1-2-3, I thought for a minute that I was watching a TV show teaching me how to count. I fumbled for the remote, but when I punched the power button, there was Julia Child cooking in the kitchen. And I could have sworn she had passed. It took me several minutes to figure out that the big, red numbers were on my clock. I wish I had not taken all my eye masks to share at work. Then I wouldn't have this problem. Finally, with the help of a double dose of Benadryl, I eased on back to sleep. I set my alarm to go off a little earlier than usual so that I could go to the drive-thru for breakfast to see how much money I would save with my senior discount. I guess I was more tired than I thought. The lady at the drive-thru told me they weren't serving breakfast. Then she asked me if I needed a deposit slip.

Note to self: Buy new eye mask — extra thick.

# APRIL 13

# AS LUCK WOULD HAVE IT

Oh no! It is Friday the 13th! Not that I am superstitious or anything, but I can't be too careful, especially since I'm getting older. I like the saying, "older and wiser," so I should do my best to act the part, right? I got up slowly and walked gingerly into the kitchen to make coffee. It took me a little longer than usual. It's hard to make coffee with your fingers crossed. As I got ready for the day, I decided to avoid wearing makeup since there was a chance that I would drop my compact with the crossed-fingers thing going on. I certainly did not want the mirror to crack. As I headed for the car to visit some more stores with senior discounts, I spotted a black cat running across the driveway. I stopped dead in my tracks. I immediately reached in my purse and got out a penny. I tossed it on the sidewalk in front of me and then picked it up as I strolled to the car. Fortunately, it landed heads up. I then stopped by the park to look for a four-leaf clover. I never did find one. On the way home from Lucky's Grocery Store, I drove to a nearby restaurant and ordered carry-out for lunch. My take-out number was 13. I left without getting my food.

Note to self: Buy rabbit's foot. Order pizza delivery.

# SPACE SHOES

My feet have been killing me lately. It seems I have had a constant battle with either bunions, corns, heel pain, arch pain, or toe pain the past few months. Today, I decided to go shoe shopping because every pair of shoes I own hurts. Well, it did not take me long to figure out that the days of cute, fashionable flats and sandals were gone. And forget heels. Even a slight lift would likely make me lose my balance. Obviously, I needed more support. I ended up in an orthopedic shoe store ... and let me just say that there are no fashionable orthopedic shoes to be found. Oh, they may advertise that the industry has stepped up the fashion features and that there is no longer a need to compromise on style, but what are they supposed to say? They surely are not going to admit that their customers will look like a decrepit granny shuffling behind her walker in glorified clodhoppers. The shoes I bought claim to have space-age foam that molds to your feet with a cupping action. Well, for $175 they should be able to "send" me into space with one quick jump. And no senior discount at this store. Guess I'll just buy one pair and wear them every day.

Note to self: Buy Odor Eaters spray, powder, and insoles.

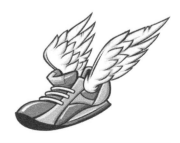

# APRIL 15

# CONFETTI

Tax deadline day — ugh! I had to go by Taxes "R" Us to sign my returns today. I'm getting back a whopping $26. It cost me more than that to get my taxes done. And by the way, no senior discount here either. I can't wait until I draw social security, then maybe I won't even have to file taxes. I don't know. I haven't opened my stack of mail that has been piling up for months from the Social Security Administration and Medicare. I've got a few months to go, so I am waiting until the last minute to read up on everything. I don't like facing reality. It is just not fun. My friends tell me that I will likely have to pay more taxes when I get older. I don't know if they are telling the truth or not. Sometimes they lie, not meaning to. Their comprehension about some things just gets a little fuzzy. The answers are lying over there on my desk somewhere, but some things I just don't want to know.

Note to self: Buy paper shredder. Out of sight, out of mind.

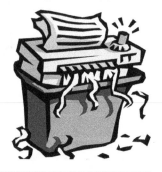

# APRIL 16

# BON VOYAGE

I have decided to put my $26 tax refund toward a cruise. I've never been on one, and I think it's about time that I had a little fun in life. I don't have that many years left. I spent all day at my travel agent's office. She didn't seem too thrilled that I was there. Maybe it was because I have been using her for years and haven't booked a trip yet. But I told her that this time I really was going somewhere. I finally decided on a Carnival cruise because I liked the name. It sounded like the most fun. Then I picked the ship that I wanted to go on. I picked the Elation. I haven't had that feeling in a long time. After a long look at the pictures of the towel animals to confirm that I made the best choice, my travel agent suggested that I get a room without a balcony so that I couldn't fall off into the ocean. She also said that I would need to wear a life vest 24/7, just in case I was thrown overboard in rough waters. I told her as I left that I would need to think about it some more.

Note to self: Book enclosed, glass-bottom boat tour at Silver Springs. Buy life vest.

APRIL 17

# MEMORY JOG

This afternoon, I contemplated ordering a new magazine subscription. I'm getting bored with reading my large-print Reader's Digest. I just need a change. Plus, I would prefer more pictures and less reading. We old farts not only need to know about practical advice and medical breakthroughs, but we also need to know that things in our past have not been forgotten, literally. If my memory keeps fading as quickly as it has been lately, looking at pictures in a magazine may help. *Reminisce* and *Good Old Days* were my top magazine picks. *Senior Fitness* and *Eating Well* did not make my list of favorites. Pictures are such a powerful means to reintroduce a blast from the past. Besides, nostalgia is important for recalling happy, personal memories. Things were just better back then. Fashions were classier, logos were timeless, things were made better, and life was simpler. Change is not always for the best. When I say to my children, "They don't make 'em like they used to," they just laugh and say, "Thank goodness!"

Note to self: Remind my children AGAIN that they don't call them "The Good Old Days" for nothing!

## APRIL 18

# COMPRESSION OBSESSION

I noticed today, as I was putting lotion on my dry, scaly legs, that my varicose veins were out of control. They looked like 3D road maps bulging and twisting all over the place. I know that I am more at risk for varicose vein issues simply because I am getting older. Imagine that. I also understand that it is a more common problem for women than men. Of course. I'm two for two. It's also hereditary. Make that three for three. I read that exercising and losing weight helps to alleviate the problem. Well, maybe, if I had a written guarantee. I can at least keep them from getting worse by resting and elevating my legs. Now that should be very doable; in fact, it sounds heavenly. I am also excited about buying some compression stockings to help the blood flow and decrease the swelling in my legs. They're easier to put on than leggings because I don't have to pull them over my hips, and the color choices are amazing. I love them all — solids, prints, plaids, stripes. I'm becoming quite the accessory fashion queen these days.

Note to self: Order compression stockings in every color and pattern. Order adjustable bed.

# EYE ON THE PRIZE

I received a letter in the mail today about my upcoming high school reunion. It's one of those cluster reunions, you know, several classes combining for one reunion. I figure this was because the numbers are dwindling, and the attendees for just one class would be too small of an event. Let's face it, many of my classmates have already kicked the bucket. I'll be curious to see who is left. It will also be fun to see who has aged gracefully and who has not. It's a good thing we wear nametags because some folks, no doubt, will not even resemble what they looked like in high school. Some will obviously look better than others. Some will have lost weight, and some will have swollen up. Some will have hair, and some will not. Some will have had lifts and tucks, and others clearly will not have. The letter said that they will be awarding a prize for the person who has changed the most. I am no longer the wallflower nerd that I was in high school. I was a late bloomer, so folks may be surprised at how good I look now. I think I may be in the running for first place.

Note to self: Make appointment with plastic surgeon and permanent makeup artist.

# THE NOD

I went to see my eye doctor again this afternoon. I am at the point where I need to get glasses because when I drop my contacts while I'm trying to put them in my eyes, I can't see to find them. Then I have no choice but to open a new pair. It is just getting too costly. As I sat down to start my eye exam, I felt very confident about passing the eye chart test. I had memorized the big "E" at the top from the last appointment, so at least I was off to a good start. I should have memorized more rows. I am now going to be wearing trifocals. I will have three differ-ent powers to correct my vision in one lens. That should be easy enough to adjust to — if I don't have to move my head! When I do get brave enough to move my head, I will probably look like a bobblehead nodding my head up and down trying to figure out which part of the lens I am supposed to look through. It makes me dizzy just thinking about it. And it's scary to think what I may be nodding "yes" to. Could be interesting. Well, at least it will be fun to sport some fashionable frames. Elton John will have nothing on me!

Note to self: Buy extra strength nausea medicine.

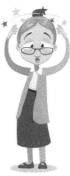

## APRIL 21

# THE LAYERED LOOK

With summer approaching, a friend of mine and I decided to go into town today to shop for new summer dresses. We checked to see which stores offered senior discounts, and off we went. The colors this year are so pretty, and there were ample bright patterns to choose from. We both got an armful of dresses and went to the dressing rooms to try them on. The sizes have obviously gotten smaller, so we had to go back and forth from the dressing rooms to the racks to find bigger ones. After what seemed like hours, we both got lucky and found a dress we liked. We checked out at the register and headed to the car feeling like fashionistas. Just as we were walking out the door, the alarm went off and nearly scared the pee out of us. It was so loud! The manager came running after us and yelled for us to stop. We eased back into the store so he could check our bags. Fortunately, our receipts were in the bags also. We once again headed out the door and the alarm went off again. As it turned out, Edith had accidentally put her own clothes back on over one of the dresses she had tried on.

Note to self: Call friends and neighbors to collect Edith's bail.

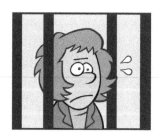

# APRIL 22

# UNDONE

I was still excited about the new dress I bought yesterday, and I could not wait to wear it. I had not bought a new dress in a long time. I got up extra early so that I wouldn't have to hurry to get ready for church. After showering, I slipped my new dress over my head and finished primping in the mirror. Off to church I went. I sat on the back row in case I needed to pee during the service. Then I could come and go without making a spectacle of myself. I hate to be the center of attention. Toward the end of the service, we were led by the usher to the front of the church to take communion. As we made our way up the aisle, the pianist began playing "Just as I Am." We joined in with the congregation and began singing the old classic hymn, and about that time, the lady behind me started snickering and finished buttoning up my dress. Now I remember why I never buy dresses.

Note to self: Donate new dress to Goodwill. Order more elastic pants and pullover tops.

# GUT DECISION

**B**etween Edith's unintentional shoplifting episode and my church episode, I decided to educate myself on memory supplements. Loss of brain power can be just downright humiliating. Once again, I read up on yet another subject that affects senior citizens. This trying to stay informed garbage is exhausting, and honestly it is getting old. But I like to be "in the know." I read about numerous supplements to help with focus and concentration. There was everything from Ginkgo Biloba to B12 . . . and a million more that I couldn't even pronounce. As I read further, I learned that it is generally more advisable just to exercise, eat lots of veggies, nuts, whole grains, olive oil, fish and poultry. So I should forget the supplements? I think I remember reading somewhere that it is good for your health to drink a daily glass of wine. Sounds like a good idea to me. Yes, I will forget the supplements. I have a good feeling about this. I think I'll just go with my gut on this one.

Note to self: Buy biggest wine glass I can find . . . or maybe a carafe.

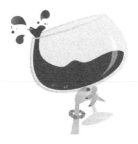

# APRIL 24

# VERY SMART PHONE

I am so excited! I finally entered the 21st century and bought myself a smart phone. I got the one with the big screen — a plus-size I think they call it. I picked neon pink so that I can find it easily. It is thrilling to finally own one . . . but I will be even more delighted when I learn how to use the confounded thing! The capabilities seem limitless. The salesman told me that I can check the date, time, weather, make calls, and take pictures. Just hope I can remember my passcode. It's a good thing that the little picture things (I think they call them acorns) have labels so I can tell what button to push. It even has a compass in case I get lost. I have a few friends in my contact list already. The touch screens are so sensitive. I have accidentally called someone a dozen times so far. And I can't believe it works with an invisible cord. I keep forgetting that I don't have to stay seated at the kitchen table to talk.

Note to self: Practice walking and talking without a phone cord.

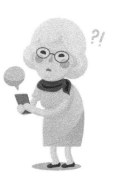

# THE PRUNE

This morning, when I looked in the mirror, I was appalled by all the wrinkles I saw. They seem to be multiplying and getting deeper by the day. Well, here I go again. Like I need to spend a few more hours of my time reading about the joys of aging. The first bit of wisdom I read was that wrinkles are a natural part of aging. Really? That was a waste of ink. I could have figured that one out. And it goes on to say that as I age, my skin will get thinner, drier, and less elastic. More waste of ink. I need solutions. After a lot of research, I found some. There is Manuka honey, olive oil, egg whites, baking soda and water, and apple cider vinegar. One article said to slice a lemon and rub on my wrinkles. I even read about how to make an avocado mask. There are also certain foods to eat with wrinkle-fighting elements — too numerous to mention. Well, I didn't know I'd have to buy out the grocery store to soften my wrinkles. This just seems like a well-planned conspiracy by the food industry. I'm not falling for it.

Note to self: Schedule Botox appointment.

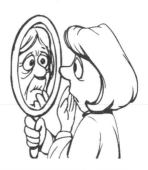

# APRIL 26

# GOBBLE, GOBBLE

Flab, flab, flab. It's disgusting! The flab around my middle I can disguise, and frankly I have gotten pretty good at it. My double chin is another story. Turtlenecks in the winter are great, but the stares I get when I wear them in the summer are a little annoying. One solution I read about was to do the "jaw jut." All I must do is tilt my head back, stare at the ceiling, push my lower jaw forward to stretch the skin under my chin, hold it for a ten-count, and repeat ten times. Well, doing face yoga to get rid of my turkey neck is not as easy as it sounds, and now my jaws are killing me. How about some home remedies for sagging skin? Sure, there are options, but they also involve going broke at the grocery store. Oils can help, and there are at least a dozen kinds that may do the trick . . . but staying slicked down and greasy is just not practical. My friend told me about a wonderful secret to shrink things, so I decided to use it on my sagging chin. Thank goodness for friends who tell secrets.

Note to self: Buy several tubes of Preparation-H.

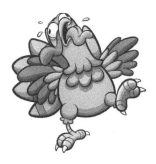

# THE ULTIMATE PLAN

I caught a segment earlier today on one of those TV morning talk shows as I was waiting to see if my double chin would shrink before my eyes. There was some financial expert talking about pre-arranged funerals. He was saying that by a certain age, which I have surpassed, everyone should have a plan in place so that our loved ones won't have the worry and financial stress of planning and paying for a funeral. Not exactly what I wanted to hear. It's not a pleasant subject. It did get me thinking, however. I'm not even sure where I want to be buried. My family may even think I want to be cremated, but the thought of me sitting in an urn on a mantle just does not seem right. What color casket do I want, and what kind of flowers? I want lots of flowers. And what songs do I want at my funeral? There are so many that I love. And what will I wear? Gosh, I don't know. I need to make some decisions and let my wishes be known. Maybe later. I've got time.

Note to self: Read books on how to increase life expectancy.

# $$ CHALLENGE

Pretty soon, I will be able to get my well-deserved social security check, finally! I am simply tired of working, and honestly, I have earned the right to get paid for being lazy. I'm pretty sure it won't be enough to live on, but I am just going to have to make it work. So, I went to the store today and bought a ledger so that I could make out a budget. Okay ... each month, I have a mortgage payment, groceries, utilities, cable bill, phone bill, insurance, and church offering. Plus, I will need to allow for extra stuff like gifts, doctor appointments, car repairs, entertainment, and vacations. Hmm, it's much worse than I thought. Either the calculator is on the fritz, or my financial forecast is very gloomy. I will just need to cut back, that's all. Eat less, go less, give less, shower less, turn up the thermostat, use candles, and stay well.

Note to self: Throw ledger in firepit, and borrow money from the kids.

# THE FAIR PRIZE

The county fair is in town this week. I always did enjoy the sights and sounds of the midway, so a few of us gals decided to go, just so we could prove that we were still young enough to have fun. I could not wait to get my hands on a funnel cake covered in powdered sugar. Cotton candy was a "must" also. At least I remembered to wear elastic britches, just in case I needed a hot dog and some popcorn, too. I did. After eating, a couple of us tried our luck at the coin toss with the anticipation of bringing home a giant teddy bear. I even rubbed my sticky fingers on the coin, hoping it would stick to the plate. No luck. I think the game was rigged. So, we moved on to the basketball throw and then to the little, floating ducks target game. Still no stuffed animal. No prize whatsoever. Not even a goldfish. After getting lost in the house of mirrors, we finally made it out and decided to ride some rides. The Tilt-A-Whirl was first. We laughed so hard as we were spinning non-stop. We had to leave after that. Imogene was nauseous, and Gertrude wet her Depends . . . and they apparently were not very dependable.

Note to self: Buy goldfish at the pet store and brag about winning it at the fair.

# PARTY HEARTY

I am planning a surprise party for my friend who is turning 80. I've got to decide on games, food, and entertainment. It's a big milestone, so I want it to be a special celebration. I have gotten all kinds of suggestions from my friends. Pin the tail on the donkey, drop the clothespin in the bottle, ring toss, musical chairs, and indoor balloon volleyball were all mentioned as games that we should play. We also discussed what kind of drinks would go best with pureed foods. Boost milkshakes could work. A cake with 80 candles may be too hard to blow out, but we all could help. I checked the date on my fire extinguisher, and we're good to go. But when I stopped to really think about all this, the party sounded way too boring. I refuse to act my age, and I try my best to make sure others don't either. We are never too old to have fun, so let the new party plans begin.

Note to self: Buy Spin the Bottle game. Order Ex-Lax cake with trick candles that cannot be blown out. Check price for male stripper.

# MAY 1

# E-I-E-I-O

I've recently joined a community choir because I love to sing, and it gives me something to do. I used to be a soprano, but after having kids, I became an alto. I am still trying to figure out why. Probably all the yelling. With the hormone changes, or whatever else is going on with my body now that I have hit old age, I now sound more like a bass. My range used to be nearly two octaves, but now it's about five notes. I guess before too long, I will become a monotone, which I will proudly rename a "one-note wonder." I may be the first one ever to be blackballed from a volunteer membership organization. However, I'm not the only one that is struggling. My new elderly ladies' choir has an array of voices that sound like croaking toads, screeching owls, and every animal in between. Good thing our director chose a repertoire of animal sound songs. Between our jungle noises, farm animal sounds, and the clatter of our rhythm band accompaniment, we shouldn't have to worry too much about hitting the correct notes.

Note to self: As advertising chairman, remind the public that the choir concert has now become a free event and that earplugs are available.

# MAY 2

# THE NAME GAME

The "golden years" — the beginning of age-imposed physical, emotional, and cognitive limitations. And they call them golden years, why? The word "golden" is associated with bright, shining, lustrous, rich, flourishing, valuable, precious, and prosperous. Who came up with the term anyway? I don't like misconceptions and misleading phrases. I think it is just society's way of trying to make us feel better about ourselves. I have also heard this stage of life referred to as the "twilight years" and the "sunset years." As the names would indicate, I am not exactly entering the prime of my life. So, who are they fooling? Not me. It's time to rename this distinct and special life state, so I am taking the bull by the horns. I call it like I see it. A more accurate term would be "diminished then finished" or maybe "the downturn to crash and burn." "Highway to decay" is rather catchy, too. I'll leave the final selection to the professionals.

Note to self: Contact Merriam-Webster about renaming the "golden years."

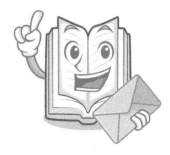

## MAY 3

# A MATTER OF OPINION

This morning, as I was sipping on my Bloody Mary and eating my ice cream, I read up on the secrets of staying young. Part of staying healthy is to eat a good diet. Fortunately, opinions matter. My breakfast was more than good. It tasted fantastic. Included in the article was a list of the greatest 25 super foods. Unfortunately, I only like about five or six of them. One of them I have never even heard of. The list is just truly not practical. Blueberries stain my teeth, strawberry seeds get stuck in my teeth, and garlic breath will make me lose friends. Salmon, beets, and ginger just taste nasty. Beans and broccoli will also make me lose friends, for a different reason. Greek yogurt and green tea are two things on the list that I could only ingest if it were a matter of life and death. And chia seeds? As in chia pet? Not this lady! Well, at least my trip to the grocery store today will be a short one.

Note to self: Buy case of Ensure to use as chasers.

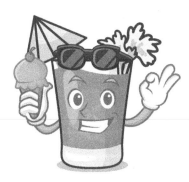

# MAY 4

# BIKE TO TRIKE

I woke up to an unusually beautiful day, so I decided that I would get my bicycle out of the shed and ride it around the neighborhood. The tires were not completely dry rotted yet, so I just had to knock off the spider webs, and I was ready to ride. I wore some old clothes so that the rust would not ruin my outfit. I took off down the sidewalk, and after only two falls, I got the hang of it again rather quickly. When I met up with someone walking on the sidewalk, all I had to do was ring my little bell and toot my little horn, and they got out of my way. It was invigorating to get some fresh air and exercise. After nearly making it to the end of the street, I was getting out of breath, so I headed back to the house. About that time, a car whizzed past me and scared me half to death. He didn't even slow down. As I turned to make an obscene gesture, I ran into my neighbor's mailbox. No broken bones. I had my rabbit's foot in my pocket.

Note to self: Buy jumbo, neon tricycle with a flag on it. Buy new mailbox for neighbor.

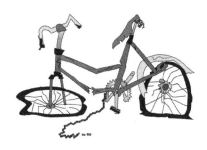

## MAY 5

# MI ESPAÑOL

W̲e observe Cinco de Mayo on this day each year. Celebrations will go on all over the U.S. commemorating the Mexican Army's victory over the French Empire on this day in 1862. Parades, food, music, dancing. Salsa, taquitos, tostados, sangria, and margaritas. It doesn't get much better than that. My friends and I are heading downtown this afternoon to join in the festivities. I even bought a new sombrero and a bright red Mexican skirt to wear. I can't wait to dance when the mariachi band gets fired up. It has been so long since I have been out on the town to have fun. I'm going to let loose. I can't wait to show everyone that party skills do not have to decline with age. I am going to take my maracas and castanets to add a little life to the party when I dance and sing to, "La Cucaracha." I also will be practicing my favorite Spanish sentence, "Uno, dos, tres Margaritas!"

Note to self: Remember the saying, "One tequila, two tequila, three tequila — floor!"

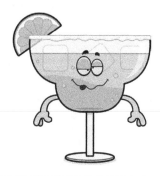

# MAY 6

# PUZZLED

The weather today was yucky. I decided to stay indoors and work on a jigsaw puzzle since I was feeling a bit under the weather. As it turned out, I could count higher in Spanish than I thought . . . so I certainly was not up to any physical or mental challenge. I looked through my closet and selected one of my favorite puzzles and then set up the card table on my sun porch so that I could watch the rain. The puzzle was a beautiful seascape. After finding my corner pieces, I laid out all the other pieces and set the box upright so that I could easily see the picture. It did not help. Most of the pieces were the same color, in slightly different shades. That is not fair. So, I had to rely on the shapes of the pieces. Well, that did not help either. The shapes were almost all the same. After a few hours, I only had a few pieces connected, and my head was killing me. I ended up forcing a few of the pieces to fit, just so it looked as though I had accomplished something. How lame to have to cheat on a jigsaw puzzle. It seems that the older I get, the more my skills vanish into thin air.

Note to self: Buy an easy, multi-colored, extra-large piece jigsaw puzzle. Order book: *How to Cheat at Nearly Everything.*

# PICTURE PERFECT

After dreaming last night that my family burned all of my pictures when I died, I decided that I needed to schedule a photographer to take a new family portrait, just in case it was a premonition . . . and just in case my book on how to increase life expectancy failed. I looked up several local photographers and called them to get prices and availability. Highway robbery! They are just a little too proud of their talent. They could go out and buy a fancy, new camera for the price they are asking for taking a few measly pictures. I finally found one that was reasonable, so I booked Cheap Shots. The whole family will be here for the photo shoot next week. We will be dressed in color-coordinated outfits and photographed in my back yard. I want to be remembered as a beautiful, young-looking grandma that will have everyone asking my grandkids, "Is that really your grandmother?" That is, if they don't place me behind a branch of the weeping willow tree.

Note to self: Have weeping willow tree removed. Pay extra for super-duper retouching.

# S-T-R-E-T-C-H-E-D TO THE LIMIT

As I left the senior center this afternoon, I saw a poster about a water aerobics class that would be offered soon. It advertised that it was a great form of low-impact exercise that was easier on the joints. I found out that a couple of my friends were going, so I figured that I would give it a try. I stopped by the desk to sign up. The class would allow me to get some exercise without hurting my bad knees. Fabulous. I didn't think about the fact that I would have to go buy a swimsuit. Not so fabulous. I should have thought about that before I signed up. I got in the car, and off to the store I went. I saw no sense in delaying the inevitable. I drove downtown, went to the department store, and combed through the racks. Most of the suits wouldn't fit my big toe. There was nothing to them. I finally found some with big cups and big skirts, so I grabbed a few off the rack and went into the dressing room. After looking for hidden cameras and finding none, I stripped and wiggled my way into the stretchy, nylon, hideous pieces of cloth that made me look like a colorful blimp. What an absurd attempt to hide my nudity. I looked ridiculous! My dimpled thighs, fat rolls, and onion skin would make anyone run the other way. Why do they even use the word "slimming" on the plus-size tags? That is just plain mean. I should not have fallen for it. All I can say is, "Oink!"

Note to self: Cancel water aerobics class.

## MAY 9

# FAT-B-GONE

Ironically, I got an email first thing this morning from Plus Size Clothing entitled "Celebrate Your Curves!" It's funny how that happens. It's like cyberworld is reading my mind. Or maybe "they" know what I shopped for yesterday. Yes, "they" probably do. Scary! Well, anyway, curves are nothing to celebrate. Maybe if I were 16 years old. The word is just a nice way of saying "fat." I know women are supposed to be curvy, but only in the hips and bust. I don't believe it means the tummy, thighs, and upper arms. I used to say that I was "pleasingly plump," but now I just use the term "plump." There is nothing pleasing about my reflection in the mirror. I thought by now that modern technology would have come up with a blubber scrubber to break down some of that fatty tissue under our skin. Just scrub and watch the fat go away. What a great idea for inventors to take to the *Shark Tank*. I've always wanted to be on *Shark Tank*. Becoming an inventor at my age — why not? Oh, wait . . . another lightbulb moment. I think I'll call my invention "Fat-B-Gone."

Note to self: Call InventHelp with "Fat-B-Gone" idea. Inquire about liposuction as back-up.

# MAY 10

# JOYRIDE

Today, I went car shopping. I have always wanted a sports car, and I am not getting any younger. I probably should make this purchase while I can still get a driver's license and insurance. I just can't imagine not being able to drive. I'm all for safety, but the idea of standing on the curb waiting for the public transportation bus is not a pleasant thought. I do hope that I am at least in a wheelchair by then. That way, I can just wheel onto the platform elevator in the rear, and I won't have to fight anyone for a seat. I spent a long time at the car lot going up and down the rows looking at each car. I found a beautiful, white Nissan Z. I've always wanted one. It suits me. Besides, it would help me to maintain my "young" old lady persona . . . or maybe that is a misconception on my part. It doesn't matter. Chances are, I will at least feel the part while I am cruising around in a sports car. When I asked the salesman if I could take it for a test drive, he looked as if he'd seen a ghost and hesitated to get the keys. I told him that I was as serious as a heart attack. He promptly got the keys. We got in the car and took off for a spin around town. It was a blast. If I die tomorrow, I will die happy.

Note to self: Write thank-you notes to salesmen who helped me get out of the car. Get brochure on Lincolns.

# MAY 11

# SLIPPERY FISH

Last night, I experienced a disaster that sent me fleeing to the medical supply store today. In a diligent effort to stay safe, I had put those safety fish decals on the bottom of the shower, but it was a good idea gone bad. Apparently, I was one fish shy of a school. I was all soaped up and singing up a storm when my foot went sliding away from me, and my arms went flailing as I tried desperately to remain upright. My acrobatic routine failed. I instinctively grabbed for the shower curtain to break the fall, but it just came down on top of me, rod and all. Water was everywhere, and the wreckage looked like a twister had come through my bathroom. My back, my leg, and my elbow were not so happy about the incident either. My current state can be summed up in one word — sore! So, I put my new shower chair together and placed it in a spot where I hopefully won't drown in the deluge of water coming from the shower head. Then it dawned on me. If I am sitting, how am I supposed to wash my bottom? I'll have to stand at some point. Ugh!

Note to self: Have grab rails and shower door installed.

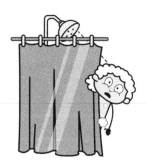

# GAS (NOT AS IN GASOLINE)

The unfortunate topic of the day is flatulence. It appears that every nook and cranny of my body is losing functionality, but who would have thought that a tiny sphincter muscle could cause such grief. If this keeps up, I will be homebound before long. I used to be able to eat anything without having to worry about my innards thundering around like an earthquake as I attempted to squelch an outwardly blast. Those inner rumblings are nothing short of painful, and the sound can usually be traced. I have become a pro at looking innocent. Recently, I thought I could get away with expelling a quiet poof of air from behind. Of course, as luck would have it, it turned out to be an "SBD" (silent but deadly). Everyone probably caught on since I was the only one not making a face and scrunching up their nose. But it's those dreaded ones that just slip out noisily with every step you take that are the most humiliating. And why is it that they always happen when everything is quiet? There was no denying the issue today when I walked by my new son-in-law as he was reading a book at my house. I just turned and said, "Welcome to the family!"

Note to self: Buy case of Gas-X . . . and a cork.

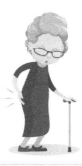

# CONVERSATION PIECES

My kids always make fun of the fact that I love trinkets. I just love little, cutesy things to put around the house. That is the main reason I need to declutter, but I love my "stuff." I hate when the girls shake their heads and say, "You need to get rid of this junk NOW so that we won't have to!" It's not that I want them to have to deal with it, but it's just that I enjoy looking at all my little dust collectors and reminiscing about the person, place, or story behind them. They make for good conversation, again and again. I realize that my trinkets may become tackier the older I get. I saw this happen to my mom. That gaudy basket of metal flowers, the gold plastic Kleenex box cover, and other such "finds" from the Dollar Tree. Yikes! My daughters recently talked me into donating some of my treasures to a local charity center. It made me sad, and it was all I could do not to go buy them back. I shudder to think of the giant bonfire that will burn in my backyard when I die. I can just envision all my trinkets crackling, melting, and withering away into ashes.

Note to self: Go shopping at local charity center and Dollar Tree. Bequeath tacky trinkets to remaining living friends.

# DISNEY CLASSICS WITH A TWIST

For some reason, my brain flashed back to a funny memory today. First off, I am grateful that I had a memory flashback at all. Any memory these days is good. One morning while sitting in church, my friend whispered in my ear for me to look around and take notice that all the old folks had big ears and big noses. She said that those two appendages never quit growing. Not a very spiritual topic, but one that was voiced and contemplated, nonetheless. After I snickered to myself, I began surveying my fellow church members in a whole new way. This piqued my curiosity. After church, I researched the issue and came to understand that what I call the "Old-Age Dumbo/Pinocchio Syndrome" is, in fact, true. The ears and nose are made of cartilage, and cartilage continues to grow. To add fuel to the fire, gravity is a contributing factor as well. As cartilage gets older, it gets thicker and less elastic, causing sagging and drooping, which makes the ears and nose appear larger. So, we old folks can not only flap our ears and fly, but we can tell a lie and get away with it.

Note to self: Request hymns for church next Sunday: "I'll Fly Away" and "I Love to Tell the Story."

# CHINNY-CHIN-CHIN

I went to visit an elderly friend of mine today in the nursing home. I try to do this occasionally because I know how much she looks forward to having company. Once I was able to get in the door, after finally remembering the correct code, I ventured down the hall of Mayberry Lane. The odor alone was enough to make me want to turn around, but I took a deep breath and held it until I reached the end of the hall. I then entered a large room. Some folks were doing puzzles, and others were watching TV. Some were just staring into space. One man seemed content to watch the fish swim around in the tank — for most of the day, from what I hear. Another gentleman was playing an out-of-tune piano and singing his heart out. I spotted my friend sitting in a chair by the window drinking a cup of coffee, talking to herself. Maybe she thought she already had company . . . I am not sure. I walked up to her and gently interrupted her "conversation." As I sat down beside her, the sun caught one side of her face just long enough for me to eye several shining, gray hairs dangling from her chin. Hmm . . . one more thing to add to the "woohoo list" of things yet to come. We had a lovely visit, despite my failed attempts to avoid periodic glimpses of her chinny-chin-chin. My only thought was, "When this happens to me, will I wax, shave, or pluck?" Well, that is the last thing I thought that I would be pondering today. Preoccupied with this newest, unsightly vision, I went home, got my magnifying mirror out, and took it over to the window to have a look. Nothing yet. Whew! I have discussed the subject with another beardless friend, and we have determined that we will take Uber to the electrolysis center if this happens to us.

Note to self: Stock up on Nair. Waxing and plucking hurt, razors leave stubbles, and Uber will probably not pick up at the nursing home.

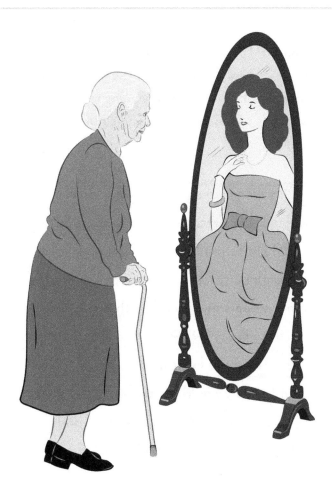

# CONCLUSION

The senior citizenship thing — I've got this!  There IS no "downhill slide" as far as I am concerned because I am going to "put it in reverse" as long as I have breath left in me.  The good Lord may have another idea, but I'm certainly going to let Him know how I feel — like He doesn't already know.  My goal is to reach 100, reign as queen of the nursing home, and give my caregivers a run for their money.

My plan is to age like a bottle of wine

And only get better with the passage of time

I will fight to the finish for senior perfection

As I continue to head in the opposite direction

From the dead-end road and that slab of stone

That will say "R.I.P. — Here Lies Joan"

I may be living in deep denial

But I simply would like to "go out" in style

It is just my nature, a matter of pride

To travel UP THE DOWNHILL SLIDE

CPSIA information can be obtained
at www.ICGtesting.com
Printed in the USA
BVHW010203020821
613401BV00003B/172

9 781649 904065